Insulin Resistance Cookbook

40 Delicious Recipes That Can Aid In Weight Loss, Reduce Insulin Resistance And Help Prevent Prediabetes

by
KATYA JOHANSSON

Copyright © 2016 by Katya Johansson.
All Rights Reserved.

More Books at www.katyajohansson.com

TABLE OF CONTENTS

INTRODUCTION 1
Breakfast recipes 3
   1. SOY ZUCCHINI NOODLES RECIPE 3
   2. PORRIDGE WITH DATES AND HONEY 4
   3. BLUEBERRY and RASPBERRY MUFFINS 6
   4. QUINOA WITH FRESH APPLE 7
   5. OVERNIGHT PROTEIN OATMEAL 8
   6. CHOCOLATE CHIA OVERNIGHT OATS 9
   7. PINEAPPLE MUESLI 10
   8. GREEN SMOOTHIE 11
   9. SCRAMBLED EGGS WITH SMOKED SALMON 12
   10. AVOCADO SMOOTHIE 14
Lunch recipes 15
   11. CHICKEN PROVENCALE CASSEROLE 15
   12. BAKED SALMON AND MUSSELS IN FOIL 17
   12. BAKED SALMON AND MUSSELS IN FOIL 17
   13. LOW CARB CASSEROLE 18
   14. CHICKEN AND ZUCCHINI 20
   15. EGGPLANT, SQUASH, AND ZUCCHINI CASSEROLE 21
   16. CABBAGE ROLLS 23
   17. STUFFED CABBAGE ROLLS 24
   18. STUFFED MUSHROOMS 26
   19. SLOW-COOKER POT ROAST 27
   20. ZUCCHINI PARMESAN 28
Dinner Recipes 29
   21. ITALIAN STYLE COD 29
   22. LAMB KEBABS 30
   23. SALMON AND BROCCOLI 32
   24. STUFFED TURKEY BREAST 33
   25. Eggplant Ratatouille 35
   26. QUICK MADE PORK 37
   27. CHICKEN AND APPLE BURGERS 38
   28. SALMON AND ASPARAGUS 40
   29. HIGH FIBER BREAD 41
   30. TILAPIA, MUSHROOM DUXELLES 43
Desserts 45
   31. MOLTEN CHOCOLATE CAKES 45

32. NO SUGAR OAT DROPS _____ 47
33. ALMOND BUTTER CHOCOLATE CHIP COOKIES _____ 49
34. CHOCOLATE PEANUT BUTTER FUDGE _____ 50
35. CARAMEL MACCHIATO CHEESECAKES _____ 51
36. CHEESE MOUSSE AND BERRIES _____ 53
37. LEMON GELATIN DESSERT _____ 54
38. STRAWBERRY COCONUT POPSICLES _____ 56
39. CHOCOLATE BLACK FOREST TRIFLE _____ 57
40. LOW-SUGAR BROWNIES _____ 58
CONCLUSION _____ 60

INTRODUCTION

Insulin is a hormone made in the pancreas, an organ located behind the stomach. Its main role is to regulate the amount of nutrients circulating in the bloodstream.
Although insulin is mostly implicated in blood sugar management, it also affects fat and protein metabolism.

Sometimes our cells stop responding to insulin like they are supposed to. In other words, they become "resistant" to the insulin.
This condition is termed insulin resistance, and is very common.

Wikipedia's definition of insulin resistance is: "Insulin resistance (IR) is generally regarded as a pathological condition in which cells fail to respond to the normal actions of the hormone insulin. The body produces insulin when glucose starts to be released into the bloodstream from the digestion of carbohydrates in the diet. Normally this insulin response triggers glucose being taken into body cells, to be used for energy, and inhibits the body from using fat as energy".

When blood sugar levels exceed a certain threshold, a diagnosis of type 2 diabetes is made. In fact, this is a simplified version of how type 2 diabetes develops. Insulin resistance is the principal cause of this common disease.

The recommended diet for this condition is: green vegetables like broccoli, zucchini, eggplant, carrots, capsicum, celery, cucumber, lettuce, tomato, onion, shallot, leeks, green beans, asparagus, bok choy, choy sum, snow peas, mushrooms, bean sprouts, alfalfa sprouts, rhubarb, leeks, chives and if you can stomach them, you can have cauliflower, Brussel sprouts and cabbage.

The list of condiments includes: soy sauce, fish sauce, oyster sauce and tomato paste, a whiff of vinegar, lemon/lime juice, mustard and Worcestershire sauce.
You can have clear soups, miso soup, stock cubes and vegetable soup.

Tomato juice is allowed, about 1/4 of a cup but only a brand that has no added sugar.

Cut down on carbs like white bread, pasta, rice, noodles, potatoes, pumpkin and sweet potatoes, kumara, turnips, corn, peas and beetroot.

Add a bean mix, cannellini beans, red kidney beans, chickpeas, hummus, quinoa, and lentils (a very small quantity) to the diet.

Once the body starts to get resistant to insulin, it can be a difficult process to reverse because of body's resistance to insulin.

Insulin resistance is a common basis for development of glucose intolerance, including diabetes and coronary artery disease, renal disease and blindness.

It is difficult to reverse this condition, but not impossible.

It is possible to reverse insulin resistance and it could take 6 months of hard work, strict diet and exercise, but as said not impossible.

Breakfast Recipes

1. Soy Zucchini Noodles Recipe

INGREDIENTS:

- 2 zucchinis, spiraled
- ½ teaspoon oil

Sauce:
- ¼ cup soy sauce
- 1 tablespoon of rice vinegar
- 1 tablespoon sesame oil
- ½ teaspoon freshly grated ginger
- toasted sesame seeds

METHOD:

1. For the sauce, combine soy sauce, rice vinegar, sesame oil and grated ginger in a bowl and mix well.
2. Heat ½ teaspoon of oil in a pan and lightly sauté the zucchini noodles for 2 minutes.
3. Remove from heat and add enough of the sauce to coat.
4. Serve hot.

5.

2. PORRIDGE WITH DATES AND HONEY

INGREDIENTS:

- 1 cup Whole Grain Teff
- 1 tablespoon cold Unsalted Butter or Coconut Oil, cut into small pieces
- 1/4 teaspoon ground Cloves
- 3 cups filtered Water
- 1/4 cup Date Pieces or pitted dates (halved crosswise)
- 1/4 teaspoon Sea Salt
- 3 tablespoons to 4 Honey, Maple Syrup or Agave, plus additional for topping
- 1/4 cup Walnuts coarsely chopped (or nut of choice; pecan, almonds, etc.)
- Yogurt, Milk or Cream (optional)

METHOD:

1. Set a heavy, 2-quart saucepan over medium heat. Add the Teff and toast, stirring frequently until the grains emit a mild, toasty aroma and begin to pop, 3 to 6 minutes. (You will notice little white dots of popped grain but may not hear the popping.)
2. Turn off the heat and stand back to avoid sputtering. Add 3 cups of boiling water, the butter, and cloves. Stir well. Turn the heat to medium, cover, and cook at a gentle boil for 10 minutes. Stir from time to time to prevent the grains from sticking to the bottom. Mash any lumps against the side of the pan.
3. Stir in the dates, salt, and honey to taste. Cover and continue cooking until the grains are tender and one

color throughout (there should be no whitish colored grain).

3. BLUEBERRY AND RASPBERRY MUFFINS

INGREDIENTS:

DRY INGREDIENTS
- 3/4 cup Whole Wheat Flour
- 3/4 cup Oat Bran
- 1/2 cup Brown Sugar
- 1 teaspoon Baking Powder (aluminum free)
- 1/2 teaspoon Baking Soda

WET INGREDIENTS
- 1 8oz container organic Blueberry Yogurt
- 1 Egg
- 2 tablespoon. Coconut Oil
- 1/2 teaspoon Vanilla
- 1 cup frozen blueberries
- 1 cup frozen raspberries

METHOD:

1. Combine dry ingredients in a bowl.
2. Combine wet ingredients in another bowl.
3. Combine wet with dry and frozen berries.
4. Combine just until all ingredients are well mixed
5. Bake at 400 degrees for 18 minutes.

4. QUINOA WITH FRESH APPLE

INGREDIENTS:

- 1 cup hot cooked quinoa
- 1/2 unpeeled cubed apple (pink lady, honeycrisp or Fuji)
- 1/4 cup raw almonds
- 1/8 cup raisins
- 1/8-1/4 cup plain almond milk
- 1 tablespoon coconut oil
- Dash of cinnamon
- Drizzle of raw agave syrup

METHOD:

1. Stir all together and eat.

5. OVERNIGHT PROTEIN OATMEAL

INGREDIENTS:

- 3/4 cup unsweetened almond milk (or milk of choice)
- 1/2 cup Plain low fat Greek yogurt (or mashed banana, applesauce or pumpkin)
- 1/2 cup Grated carrots
- 1/4 teaspoon Salt (or to taste)
- 1/2 teaspoon Cinnamon
- 1/2 teaspoon Apple pie spice
- 2 tablespoon Baking stevia (or 1/4 cup sweetener)
- 1 cup Old Fashioned Oats
- 1/4 cup Protein powder (or additional oats)
- Optional: Toppings of choice

METHOD:

1. In a small bowl, mix all of the ingredients together.
2. Divide between 2 small bowls, mugs, or mason jars.
3. Cover and refrigerate overnight (or for at least an hour (or more) so the oats soften and absorb the liquid).
4. Top with chopped nuts, cinnamon, low sugar syrup, or vanilla Greek yogurt if desired.
5. Enjoy cold, or microwave for 30-60 seconds to enjoy warm.

6. CHOCOLATE CHIA OVERNIGHT OATS

INGREDIENTS:

- 2 cups old fashioned oats
- 2 cups milk of your choice (I used soy milk)
- ¼ cup raw cacao powder or cocoa powder
- ¼ cup pure maple syrup
- 3 tablespoons chia seeds

METHOD:

1. In a medium bowl, whisk all ingredients together until well combined.
2. Divide into smaller containers such as mason jars, cover and place in refrigerator overnight.
3. Top with fresh fruit and enjoy!

7. PINEAPPLE MUESLI

INGREDIENTS:

- 3/4 cup pistachios, shells removed and coarsely chopped
- 1/3 cup, unsweetened, flaked coconut
- 1 cup old-fashioned rolled oats
- 1/2 cup chopped dried pineapple
- 1/4 cup wheat bran
- 2 tablespoons chia seeds
- 2 tablespoons Stevia
- 2 tablespoons ground flax seed
- 2 tablespoons oat bran
- 1/8 teaspoon salt
- yogurt or milk, for serving

METHOD:

1. Heat a skillet over medium heat and add the pistachios.
2. Toast for a few minutes, just until slightly golden and fragrant.
3. Pour the pistachios into a large bowl.
4. Add the coconut to the same skillet over medium heat.
5. Stir and shake the pan until the coconut is slightly toasted, about 2 to 3 minutes.
6. Add the coconut to the bowl.

7.

8. GREEN SMOOTHIE

INGREDIENTS:

- Water as needed
- Almond milk same amount as water
- Coconut water or fresh green juice to taste
- Spinach and kale about a handful of each
- Berries of your choice (about a handful)

ENERGETIC ADD-ONS:
Coconut oil
Ground flax seeds or Chia seeds
Protein powder
Almond butter

METHOD:

1. Add the basic ingredients to you blender and blend until liquefied.
2. How much and how long depends on your blender's power and settings.
3. The best blender is the Blend Tec blender that has a perfect "Smoothie" setting.
4. Next, blend again.
5. Lastly add any more liquid or ice, as desired and blend again, if necessary.

9. SCRAMBLED EGGS WITH SMOKED SALMON

INGREDIENTS:

- 2 eggs
- 1 tablespoon coconut butter
- 1 tablespoon soy milk
- 2 ounces smoked salmon
- Chopped herbs
- Salt and pepper to taste

METHOD:

1. Crack 2 eggs into a small mixing bowl and whisk.
2. Heat a heavy-bottomed nonstick sauté pan over medium-low heat.
3. Add a tablespoon of olive oil or coconut butter.
4. Add a tablespoon of milk to the eggs and season to taste with salt and pepper.
5. Whisk thoroughly to incorporate a bit of air into the mixture.
6. Pour into hot oil or butter and let the eggs cook for up to a minute without stirring to the bottom set.
7. With a rubber spatula, gently push one edge of the egg into the center of the pan, while tilting the pan to allow the still liquid egg to flow in underneath.
8. Repeat with the other edges, until the raw egg is gone.
9. Turn off the heat and continue gently stirring and turning the egg until all the uncooked parts become firm.
10. Don't break up the egg, though. Try to keep the curds as large as possible.
11. Add an ounce or two of smoked salmon and chopped herbs.

12. Transfer to a plate when the eggs are set but still moist and soft.
13. Eggs are delicate, so they'll continue to cook for a few moments after they're on the plate.

10. AVOCADO SMOOTHIE

INGREDIENTS:

- ½ ripe avocado
- 1 ripe banana
- ½ cup low-fat yogurt
- ½ cup orange juice
- Optional: handful of ice

METHOD:

1. Combine ingredients into blender and mix well.

Lunch Recipes

11. CHICKEN PROVENCALE CASSEROLE

INGREDIENTS:

- 300g lean chicken breast, cut into chunks
- 2 tablespoons olive oil
- 2 cloves garlic, minced
- 2 cloves garlic, peeled and whole
- 2 large zucchinis, halved lengthways and cut into chunks
- 6 mushrooms, quartered
- 6 pitted black olives
- 1 small onion chopped
- ½ cup chicken stock
- 1 cup tomato sauce
- 2 spring fresh thyme
- 1 spring tarragon
- 1 spring rosemary
- Handful basil leaves
- Chopped parsley for garnish

METHOD:

1. In an oven proof casserole dish, brown the chicken in olive oil then put aside.
2. In the same casserole dish, lightly sauté the onion, zucchini, mushrooms and minced garlic in olive oil.
3. Add the tomato sauce, chicken stock and herbs.
4. Cover and cook in 160C oven for 30 minutes.
5. Remove cover and cook for another 10 minutes.

6. To serve, sprinkle with chopped parsley.

12. BAKED SALMON AND MUSSELS IN FOIL

INGREDIENTS:

- 2 x 150g salmon fillet
- 2 teaspoons of olive oil
- Salt and pepper
- 1 zucchini, cut thin lengthwise
- 4 large leaves of bok choy
- 4 black mussels
- 2 cherry tomatoes, halved

METHOD:

1. Preheat oven to 160C.
2. On a large piece of foil, layer the ingredients in the following order: zucchini, bok choy, salmon fillet, salt and pepper, bok choy again, black mussels, cherry tomatoes.
3. Bring the edges of the foil together to form a closed parcel.
4. Bake in the oven for 15 mins.

13. LOW CARB CASSEROLE

INGREDIENTS:

- ½ carrot, cut into thin strips
- ½ zucchini, cut into thin strips
- 2 mushrooms, thinly sliced
- Handful of baby spinach
- 2 shallots cut into thin strips
- 2 strips of dried seaweed cut into thin strips
- ¼ cup cauliflower rice

TO COOK VEGETABLES:
- Sesame oil
- Soy sauce
- Toasted sesame seeds

BULGOGI MARINADE:
- 2 tablespoon soy sauce
- 1 tablespoon sesame oil
- 1 tablespoon Korean chili paste
- 200 g beef, thinly sliced
- 1 egg yolk

METHOD:

1. Cut meat into thin strips and marinade in Bulgogi sauce.
2. Prepare all vegetables.
3. Cook rice and keep warm.
4. Prepare cauliflower rice.
5. Heat a little amount of sesame oil in pan, add each vegetable with a dash of soy sauce and cook on gentle heat for 2-3 minutes.
6. Set aside separately and keep warm.

INSULIN RESISTANCE COOKBOOK

7. Heat a little vegetable oil in a pan and stir fry the beef then keep warm.
8. Add a little amount of sesame oil to the same pan and cook rice for 2-3 minutes.
9. Assemble dish: add a little sesame oil on bottom.
10. Top with rice.
11. Add cooked vegetables and meat like spokes of a bicycle wheel.
12. Sprinkle with sesame seeds.
13. Carefully add the egg yolk in the middle.
14. Serve with a side of hot sauce.
15. To serve, mix all together.

14. CHICKEN AND ZUCCHINI

INGREDIENTS:

- 3 medium zucchini, sliced
- 12 ounces chicken breast or tenderloin, chopped
- 1 tablespoon garlic, finely chopped
- 1 tablespoon onion, chopped
- 2 cups sliced mushrooms
- 1/3 cup grated parmesan cheese

METHOD:

1. Spray a skillet or frying pan with cooking spray and turn to medium/high heat.
2. Add onions and garlic, sauté until they begin to turn golden brown.
3. Add the mushrooms and zucchini.
4. Sauté until mushrooms and zucchini start to become tender.
5. Add chicken and continue to sauté on high heat until chicken is completely cooked.
6. Add the parmesan cheese, stirring frequently and coating all the pieces.
7. Remove from heat once cheese has coated all pieces and melted.

INSULIN RESISTANCE COOKBOOK

15. EGGPLANT, SQUASH, AND ZUCCHINI CASSEROLE

INGREDIENTS:

- 1.5 Yellow Squash, cut into 1/2" slices
- 1 Medium Zucchini, cut into 1/2" slices
- 5 Medium Eggplants, cut into 1" cubes
- 5 Medium Yellow Onion, chopped
- 2 cloves of Garlic, minced
- 1 10oz can of Rotel (or any other diced tomatoes with chilies)
- 5 cup Canned Diced Tomatoes
- 5 cup grated Parmesan cheese
- 5 cup shredded 2% Mexican Blend cheese
- Butter Flavored Non-Fat Cooking Spray
- Garlic Salt
- Pepper

METHOD:

1. I cooked this in a toaster oven.
2. Preheat oven to 400.
3. Line a baking dish with foil and spray with cooking spray to prevent sticking.
4. Heat large nonstick skillet over medium heat.
5. When skillet is hot, coat with cooking spray.
6. Add onions and garlic.
7. Sautee until soft.
8. Add Rotel, diced tomatoes, eggplant, squash, and zucchini to pan.
9. Sprinkle with garlic salt and pepper to taste.
10. Sautee for 5 minutes.

11. Layer the eggplant/squash mixture and Parmesan, alternating until eggplant mixture is gone.
12. Top with remaining Parmesan or and the Mexican blend cheese.
13. Bake for 20 minutes (or until veggies are cooked to desired doneness).

16. CABBAGE ROLLS

INGREDIENTS:

- 1 medium head cabbage
- 1 1/2 cups uncooked white rice
- 2 tablespoons coconut butter
- 1 Onion, chopped
- Salt and pepper to taste
- 1 (46 fluid ounce) can tomato juice

METHOD:

1. Preheat oven to 325 degrees F (165 degrees C).
2. Grease a 2 quart casserole dish.
3. Steam the whole head of cabbage until it is al dente.
4. Meanwhile, in a saucepan bring 3 cups of water to a boil.
5. Add rice and stir.
6. Reduce heat, cover and simmer for 20 minutes.
7. Melt butter in a small skillet over medium heat.
8. Sauté onion until translucent; stir into cooked rice.
9. Season with salt and pepper to taste.
10. Cut the leaves off of the cabbage and cut the larger leaves in half.
11. Spoon 1 tablespoon of rice into a leaf and roll tightly.
12. Place rolls in prepared casserole dish, stacking in layers.
13. Pour tomato juice over the rolls, using enough just to cover.
14. Cover and bake in preheated oven for 2 hours.

17. STUFFED CABBAGE ROLLS

INGREDIENTS:

- 1 pound ground beef
- 1/2 pound ground pork
- 1 1/2 cups cooked rice
- 1 teaspoon finely chopped garlic
- 1 teaspoon salt, plus more to taste
- 1/4 teaspoon ground black pepper, plus more to taste
- 3 (10.75 ounce) cans condensed tomato soup
- 2 (12 fluid ounce) cans tomato juice, or more to taste
- 1/2 cup ketchup

METHOD:

1. Bring a large pot of lightly salted water to a boil.
2. Place cabbage head into water, cover pot, and cook until cabbage leaves are slightly softened enough to remove from head, 3 minutes.
3. Remove cabbage from pot and let cabbage sit until leaves are cool enough to handle, about 10 minutes.
4. Remove 18 whole leaves from the cabbage head, cutting out any thick tough center ribs. Set whole leaves aside.
5. Chop the remainder of the cabbage head and spread it in the bottom of a casserole dish.
6. Melt butter in a large skillet over medium-high heat.
7. Cook and stir onion in hot butter until tender, 5 to 10 minutes. Cool.
8. Stir onion, beef, pork, rice, garlic, 1 teaspoon salt, and 1/4 teaspoon pepper together in a large bowl.
9. Preheat oven to 350 degrees F (175 degrees C).
10. Place about 1/2 cup beef mixture on a cabbage leaf.

INSULIN RESISTANCE COOKBOOK

11. Roll cabbage around beef mixture, tucking in sides to create an envelope around the meat.
12. Repeat with remaining leaves and meat mixture.
13. Place cabbage rolls in a layer atop the chopped cabbage in the casserole dish; season rolls with salt and black pepper.
14. Whisk tomato soup, tomato juice, and ketchup together in a bowl.
15. Pour tomato soup mixture over cabbage rolls and cover dish wish aluminum foil.
16. Bake in the preheated oven until cabbage is tender and meat is cooked through, about 1 hour.

18. STUFFED MUSHROOMS

INGREDIENTS:

- 48 fresh whole baby portabella or white mushrooms (1 1/2 to 2 inches in diameter)
- 1 package (8 oz.) cream cheese, softened
- 1 box (9 oz.) frozen chopped spinach, thawed, squeezed to drain
- 1 cup freshly grated Parmesan cheese
- 1/2 teaspoon salt
- 1/4 teaspoon freshly ground black pepper
- 1/8 teaspoon ground red pepper (cayenne)
- 1/2 cup panko crispy bread crumbs
- 2 tablespoons butter melted

METHOD:

1. Heat oven to 350°F.
2. Remove stems from mushroom caps; reserve caps.
3. Discard stems.
4. In large bowl, mix cream cheese, spinach, 1/2 cup of the Parmesan cheese, the salt and both peppers until well blended.
5. Spoon into mushroom caps, mounding slightly.
6. Place mushrooms in ungreased 17x12-inch half-sheet pan.
7. In small bowl, mix remaining 1/2 cup Parmesan cheese, the bread crumbs and butter.
8. Sprinkle bread crumb mixture over filled mushroom caps, pressing lightly.
9. Bake 20 to 22 minutes or until thoroughly heated.
10. Serve immediately.

19. SLOW-COOKER POT ROAST

INGREDIENTS:

- 8 small red potatoes cut in half
- 3-pound beef boneless arm roast, trimmed of fat
- 2 tablespoons all-purpose flour
- 1 pound baby-cut carrots
- 1 jar (16 ounces) Old El Paso Thick 'n Chunky salsa

METHOD:

1. Place potatoes in 3 1/2- to 4-quart slow cooker.
2. Coat beef with flour; place on potatoes.
3. Arrange carrots around beef.
4. Pour salsa over all.
5. Cover and cook on low heat setting 8 to 10 hours.
6. Remove beef from cooker; place on cutting board.
7. Pull beef into serving pieces, using 2 forks.
8. To serve, spoon sauce over beef and vegetables.

20. ZUCCHINI PARMESAN

INGREDIENTS:

- 1 cup sliced zucchini
- 1 tablespoon shredded Parmesan cheese
- 10 squirts butter spray

METHOD:

1. Line a cookie sheet with aluminum foil, then coat with some cooking spray.
2. Place the zucchini slices out on the pan, then spritz with them with the butter spray.
3. Sprinkle on the parmesan cheese and then pop it in the oven.
4. Broil for a few minutes - until the cheese starts to brown.
5. Enjoy it while it's warm!

Dinner Recipes

21. Italian Style Cod

INGREDIENTS:

- 400g cod fillets
- 2 tablespoon grated Pecorino Romano cheese
- 2 tablespoon grated Parmesan cheese
- 2 cloves of garlic, crushed
- 50g butter, melted
- 1 tablespoon fresh parsley, finely chopped
- Salt and pepper to taste

METHOD:

1. Preheat the oven to Gas Mark 6 or 200°C.
2. Lightly grease an ovenproof dish.
3. Mix the cheeses, garlic and seasoning in a bowl.
4. Place the fillets in the ovenproof dish and cover with the cheese mixture and parsley.
5. Season to taste.
6. Bake for 15 minutes and serve immediately.

22. LAMB KEBABS

INGREDIENTS:

KEBAB MIX

- 400g minced lamb
- 2 teaspoon. garlic, peeled and finely chopped
- 2 teaspoon. ginger, peeled and finely chopped
- 1 large onion, peeled and finely chopped
- 2 teaspoon ground coriander
- 2 teaspoon ground cumin
- ¼ teaspoon ground black pepper
- 1 tablespoon fresh coriander, finely chopped
- 4 metal skewers

GREEN SALSA MIX

- 3 spring onions, chopped
- 1 tablespoon olive oil
- 4 tomatoes, chopped roughly
- 1 tablespoon pitted olives of your choice
- 1 bunch of coriander, chopped
- 1 bunch of parsley, chopped
- Juice and grated rind of a lemon

METHOD:

1. Mix the mince, onion, ginger, garlic, coriander, cumin, pepper and salt in a mixing bowl.
2. Form 16 balls out of the mince mixture.

3. Put each ball around the tip of a metal skewer and flatten slightly.
4. Place the meatballs on a baking sheet and cover and then refrigerate them for an hour.
5. Pop all the salsa ingredients a bowl and mix together.
6. Cook the skewered lamb kebabs under a preheated grill, turning every now and again, until the lamb is cooked through.
7. This will take 15 minutes.
8. Serve hot with the salsa.

23. SALMON AND BROCCOLI

INGREDIENTS:

- 4 salmon fillets weighing 460g
- 1 head of broccoli
- 1 red chili, finely chopped
- 400ml half fat single cream
- 1 tablespoon. tomato purée
- 100g red pesto
- Freshly ground pepper to taste

METHOD:

1. Preheat the oven to Gas Mark 5 or 190°C.
2. Mix the cream, tomato puree and red pesto together.
3. Then add in the chopped red chili.
4. Place the broccoli and the salmon in the red pesto sauce in 4 individual pot pie dishes, ensuring the fish is fully coated, and bake in the preheated oven for 20 minutes.
5. Remove from the oven and allow cooling for 5 minutes or so and serve.

24. STUFFED TURKEY BREAST

INGREDIENTS:

- 2 tablespoon olive oil
- 2 medium onions
- 6 garlic cloves, finely chopped
- Salt and pepper to season
- 6 x 200g turkey breasts (opt for a thicker breast in order to fillet it easier)
- 180g cheddar cheese, grated
- 100g gruyere cheese, grated
- 12 slices Parma ham
- Steamed broccoli and cauliflower
- Juice of a lemon

METHOD:

1. Pour a tablespoon of olive oil into a saucepan and place over a medium heat until the oil warms up.
2. Sauté the onions for around 4 minutes, add the garlic and cook for another 2 minutes.
3. Season the mixture with salt and pepper, then set it aside to cool down.
4. Partly fillet the turkey breast.
5. You should open up the turkey enough to make a small pocket and then stuff the cheddar and gruyere inside that pocket.
6. Season the turkey breasts with salt and pepper, and wrap two slices of Parma ham around each breast.
7. Drizzle the turkey breasts with the rest of the olive oil and bake at 180°c or Gas Mark 4 for 25 minutes,

ensuring that the ham is crispy and the chicken is fully cooked.
8. To test if the turkey is cooked, stick a skewer in it: when it comes out, the juice should be clear and not be at all pink.
9. Serve along with steamed broccoli and cauliflower, dressed with some lemon juice.

25. Eggplant Ratatouille

INGREDIENTS:

- 2 tablespoons extra virgin olive oil
- 2 onions chopped
- 4 cloves garlic minced
- 2 eggplants peeled in strips and cut into 3/4 inch cubes
- 4 zucchini cut into 1 inch cubes
- Salt and pepper to taste
- 3 bell peppers red or yellow (ribs and seeds removed, cut into 3/4 inch cubes)
- 1 can diced tomatoes
- 1 teaspoon dried thyme
- 1/2 cup basil chopped

METHOD:

1. In a large pot with a snug-fitting lid), heat oil over medium heat.
2. Cook onions and stir occasionally until soft, about 5 minutes.
3. Add garlic; cook until aromatic, about 1 minute.
4. Stir in eggplant and zucchini; season with salt and pepper to taste.
5. Add 3/4 cup water; cover, and simmer until vegetables begin to soften, stirring once, about 5 minutes.
6. Add bell peppers, stir; simmer and cover until softened, 5 minutes.
7. Stir in tomatoes and thyme; bring to a boil.
8. Reduce heat to medium-low.
9. Partially cover; simmer, until vegetables are tender (stirring often), about 15 to 20 minutes.

10. Remove from heat.

INSULIN RESISTANCE COOKBOOK

26. QUICK MADE PORK

INGREDIENTS:

- tablespoon water
- 1 tablespoon Worcestershire sauce for chicken
- 1 teaspoon lemon juice
- 1 teaspoon Dijon-style mustard
- 4 3 - ounces boneless pork top loin chops, cut 3/4 to 1 inch thick
- 1/2-1 teaspoon lemon-pepper seasoning
- 1 tablespoon butter or margarine
- 1 tablespoon snipped fresh chives, parsley, or oregano

METHOD:

1. For sauce, in a small bowl stir together the water, Worcestershire sauce, lemon juice, and mustard;
2. Set aside.
3. Trim fat from chops.
4. Sprinkle both sides of each chop with lemon-pepper seasoning.
5. In a 10-inch skillet melt butter over medium heat.
6. Add chops and cook for 8 to 12 minutes or until pork juices run clear (160 degrees F), turning once halfway through cooking time.
7. Remove from heat.
8. Transfer chops to a serving platter; cover with foil and keep warm.
9. Pour sauce into skillet; stir to scrape up any crusty browned bits from bottom of skillet.
10. Pour sauce over chops.
11. Sprinkle with chives.

27. CHICKEN AND APPLE BURGERS

INGREDIENTS:

BURGERS
- 1 lb. (500 g) ground chicken
- 1 large red onion, finely chopped
- ¼ cup (50 mL) plain dry bread crumbs
- 2 large green apples, such as Granny Smith (for a tart taste) or Golden Delicious (for a sweet taste), peeled and coarsely grated
- 1 tablespoon (15 mL) chopped fresh sage leaves
- 1 tablespoon (15 mL) fresh thyme leaves
- ¼ teaspoon (1 mL) salt
- ¼ teaspoon (1 mL) freshly ground black pepper

TO SERVE
- ¼ cup (50 mL) Dijon mustard
- 1 tablespoon (15 mL) honey
- 4 whole-wheat hamburger buns, split
- 6 tablespoon (90 mL) watercress sprigs

METHOD:

1. In a large bowl, place the chicken, onion, bread crumbs, apples, sage, thyme, salt and pepper. Using your hands, mix the ingredients together until the ingredients are distributed evenly throughout. Wet your hands, then divide the mixture into 4 equal portions and shape each into a burger about 4 in. (10 cm) in diameter and 1½ in.

(4 cm) thick. Chill the burgers for 1 hour to firm up the meat and make it easier to hold together while it cooks.
2. Preheat the grill or broiler to high. Place burgers on a rack about 6 in. (15 cm) from the source of heat. Grill or broil the burgers, turning them once, until they are golden brown on both sides and until they are still juicy but cooked through completely.
3. While the burgers cook, mix the mustard and honey in a small cup. On a flat surface, open the 4 buns with the soft cut sides up. Spread the honey mustard on cut sides of both the tops and bottoms of the buns. Pile one fourth of the watercress on the bottom of each bun.
4. When the burgers are ready, transfer a burger to the bottom of each bun, placing it on top of the watercress. Cover with the top of the bun and serve immediately

28. SALMON AND ASPARAGUS

INGREDIENTS:

- 4 skinless salmon fillets (about 4 oz/125 g each)
- 2 leeks, thinly sliced
- 8 oz. (250 g) asparagus spears
- 1 cup (250 mL) sugar snap peas
- 4 tablespoon (60 mL) dry white wine
- 1 cup (250 mL) reduced-sodium vegetable broth
- Salt and pepper

METHOD:

1. Run your fingertips over each salmon fillet to check for stray bones, pulling out any that remain.
2. Arrange the leeks in a single layer in the bottom of a large Dutch oven coated with cooking spray.
3. Lay the pieces of salmon on top.
4. Surround the fish with the asparagus and peas. Add the wine and broth, and season lightly with salt and pepper.
5. Place the Dutch oven over medium-high heat and bring broth to a boil, then cover with a tight-fitting lid and reduce the heat to low.
6. Cook the fish and vegetables until the salmon is pale pink all the way through and the vegetables are tender, about 12 to 14 minutes.
7. Sprinkle the chives over the salmon and serve.

29. HIGH FIBER BREAD

INGREDIENTS:

- Works in a bread machine, regular cycle.
- 1 slice = 1 Carb
- One loaf makes about 12 slices.
- 2 cups rye flour
- 2 tablespoon wheat gluten
- 1/2 cup oat bran
- 1/4 cup rolled oats
- 1/4 cup flax meal, more bran, or 9-grain cereal
- 1 tablespoon honey
- 1 tablespoon olive oil
- 1 teaspoon salt
- 1 teaspoon bread yeast
- 1 teaspoon caraway or nigella seeds for added flavor
- 1 and 1/4 cup lukewarm water

METHOD:

1. By adding the gluten, you can get away with using a much higher percentage of whole grain and fiber while still getting dough that rises in a bread machine.
2. By following a basic ratio of 2 cups whole flour (wheat, rye, oat, etc.) to 1 cup coarser ingredients (wheat, oat, or rice bran, 9 grain cereal, rolled oats, seeds, etc.) along with that extra gluten, the bread usually turns out firm and dense, but not leaden or overly dry.
3. You might need to adjust the amount of water by a tablespoon or two depending on your choice of grains.
4. The honey helps the yeast rise, so adding a bit more makes more porous bread.

5. The oil helps prevent the bread from drying out after baking, so the loaf retains a fresh texture for several days after baking.
6. If baking this by hand, knead for about 10 minutes, let rise for two hours, gently punch down, let rise again for an hour, and bake for about an hour at 350 F.

30. TILAPIA, MUSHROOM DUXELLES

INGREDIENTS:

DUXELLES:
- 1/2 lb. fresh mushrooms, finely chopped
- 1 onion, finely chopped
- 1 tablespoon olive oil
- 1/2 teaspoon salt
- 1/2 cup chicken stock
- black pepper to taste

TILAPIA:
- 1 tilapia fillet per person
- Splash of dry vermouth
- 1 clove of garlic
- 1 teaspoon olive oil
- Pinch of salt, pepper, nutmeg

METHOD:

1. Heat a large skillet on medium, spread oil onto it, then add onions and mushrooms.
2. Stir occasionally while reducing liquid out of the blend, on medium-low heat, for 30-60 minutes.
3. You don't need to attend it constantly, just make sure it doesn't brown too much or burn.
4. As the blend becomes dry, add stock and salt to taste (if stock is unsalted.)
5. Grind in some fresh pepper.

6. Continue to reduce until flavors are very concentrated, and texture becomes somewhat homogenized.
7. Set aside
8. Vegetables: before starting the fish, chop up some green winter vegetables and put them in a covered ceramic dish, for the microwave.
9. Splash with dry vermouth or white wine (or water-lemon juice mix) and microwave for a few minutes, just before serving.
10. For this dinner I used bok choy, Asparagus and Romanesco.
11. Many choices could work as accompaniment, such as spinach, broccoli, chard, etc.
12. Before serving the vegetables, sprinkle them with a good balsamic vinegar, salt and pepper.
13. Heat a large heavy skillet, with a lid nearby.
14. Finely mince a clove of garlic. Sprinkle salt and pepper over thawed tilapia fillets.
15. Spread olive oil on skillet, and place tilapia on medium-high heat for a minute or two on one side.
16. Flip the fish fillets carefully onto the other side, so as not to break them apart.
17. Toss in the garlic and wait a moment to let it sear.
18. While searing the garlic, sprinkle a tiny pinch of nutmeg or mace onto the upper side of each fillet.
19. Now add a splash of dry vermouth (or a un-oaked white wine) to deglaze the pan and prevent the garlic from burning.
20. Once the alcohol has evaporated out of the liquid (a minute or two) put the lid on the pan and reduce heat, to steam a moment while plating the rest of the meal.
21. Plate the tilapia atop a couple tablespoons of Duxelles, alongside a large pile of vegetables, and with a sprinkling of parsley and green onions.

Desserts

31. Molten Chocolate Cakes

INGREDIENTS:

- 4 tablespoon butter, plus extra for buttering ramekins
- 6 squares Lindt 85% cacao chocolate
- 1 large egg
- 1 egg yolk
- 1 tablespoon granulated erythritol
- 1 teaspoon flour

METHOD:

1. Preheat oven to 450F and butter two 4oz ramekins well.
2. Dust ramekins with cocoa powder and set aside.
3. Melt butter and chocolate together in a small bowl set over a pan of simmering water.
4. Stir until smooth.
5. In a medium bowl, beat egg, egg yolk and erythritol together until lightened in color and thickened.
6. Add chocolate mixture and mix until combined.
7. Stir in flour.
8. Divide between ramekins.
9. At this point, you could cover and chill for later, just bring back to room temperature before baking.
10. Bake 6-7 minutes.
11. Sides will be set but center will still be soft.
12. Invert onto a plate and let sit for 10 seconds or so, then lift one side of ramekin.
13. Cake will fall out onto plate.

14. Serve immediately.

32. NO SUGAR OAT DROPS

INGREDIENTS:

- 1 1/2 cups regular rolled oats (use whatever type of oats you like)
- 1 cup coconut flakes
- 1/2 teaspoon salt
- 1 teaspoon cinnamon
- 1/2 teaspoon allspice
- 1/4 cup of almond meal (or nutmeal of your choice)
- 1/2 cup mixed nuts, finely chopped
- 1 cup dried fruit (of your choice or chocolate chips or berries)
- 3 ripe bananas, mashed (or substitute applesauce, or 2 eggs)
- 1/4 cup canola oil (or oil of your choice)
- 1 teaspoon vanilla extract

METHOD:

1. Preheat oven to 175C.
2. Line baking sheet with parchment paper.
3. In a large bowl, combine rolled oats, almond meal, mixed nuts and coconut flakes. Stir in allspice and cinnamon.
4. Add dried fruit and stir until well and evenly mixed.
5. Make sure the dried fruit do not stick together in big batches.
6. In another bowl, combine canola oil, mashed banana and vanilla extract.
7. Pour wet ingredients over dry ingredients and stir until well combined.

8. Take a large cookie cutter and press gently spoonfuls of the batter into it.
9. Remove cookie cutter.
10. Or simply form balls with your hands and flatten slightly.
11. Bake for about 20 minutes or until edges are golden brown.

33. ALMOND BUTTER CHOCOLATE CHIP COOKIES

INGREDIENTS:

- 2 ripe bananas, mashed
- 1-cup natural almond butter
- 2 tablespoons real maple syrup
- 2 cups oats
- ½ teaspoon sea salt
- ½ cup dark chocolate chips

METHOD:

1. Preheat oven to 350 F
2. In a small glass bowl, mash bananas, and stir in almond butter.
3. Microwave for 30 seconds to melt the mixture, and bring out the banana flavor.
4. Stir in maple syrup.
5. In a large bowl, combine oats and sea salt.
6. Add banana mixture to oats, and stir to combine.
7. Fold in chocolate chips.
8. Line a cookie sheet with parchment paper, and spoon out cookie dough (about 2 tbsp. per cookie).
9. Bake for 10 – 15 minutes.
10. Let cool on the cookie sheet.
11. Store in the freezer.

34. CHOCOLATE PEANUT BUTTER FUDGE

INGREDIENTS:

- ¾ cup coconut oil, melted
- 2/3-cup honey
- ¾ cup cocoa powder
- ½ cup all-natural peanut butter
- 1 tablespoon vanilla extract
- ½ teaspoon sea salt

OPTIONAL ADDITIONS:
- Raw cacao nibs
- Pumpkin seeds
- Unsweetened shredded coconut
- Hemp seeds
- Walnuts
- Slivered almonds

METHOD:

1. Melt the coconut oil in a large Pyrex measuring cup.
2. Once melted, whisk in honey, cocoa powder, peanut butter, vanilla and sea salt.
3. Pour the mixture into a parchment lined loaf pan and chill in the fridge for 1-2 hours or until completely set.
4. Cut into squares, and store in the fridge or freezer.

35. CARAMEL MACCHIATO CHEESECAKES

INGREDIENTS:

FOR THE CHEESECAKES:
- 8 oz. cream cheese, softened
- 2 tablespoon unsalted butter
- 3 eggs
- 3 tablespoon Cold Brew Coffee Concentrate (or espresso)
- 1 tablespoon sugar free caramel flavored syrup see example
- ⅓ Cup granulated sugar substitute (Swerve, Splenda, Ideal, etc.)

FOR THE FROSTING:
- 3 tablespoon unsalted butter, softened
- 3 tablespoon sugar free caramel flavored syrup see example
- 2 tablespoon granulated sugar substitute (Swerve, Splenda, Ideal, etc)
- 8oz Mascarpone cheese, softened

METHOD:

1. For the cheesecakes: combine all of the cheesecake ingredients in a magic bullet or blender.
2. Blend until smooth.
3. Pour into 9 greased silicone cupcake molds, or in a cupcake pan lined with paper liners.
4. Bake at 350 degrees (F) for 15 minutes or until firm when shaken slightly.

5. Remove and chill for one hour in the freezer or at least 3 hours (preferably overnight) in the refrigerator.
6. For the frosting: cream the butter, sugar free caramel syrup, and sweetener together until fluffy.
7. At a low speed (or it will break), blend in the mascarpone until smooth.
8. Test and adjust for desired sweetness.
9. If your frosting breaks, add a few tablespoons of regular cream cheese to stabilize it.
10. Pipe or spoon onto your chilled cheesecakes before serving.

36. CHEESE MOUSSE AND BERRIES

INGREDIENTS:

- 8 ounces mascarpone cheese
- 1 cup whipping cream
- 3/4 teaspoon vanilla stevia drops
- Berries (1 pint blueberries and 1 pint strawberries)

METHOD:

1. Whip together mascarpone, cream, and sweetener in large mixing bowl with electric mixer until stiff peaks form.
2. Pipe into individual cups and layer with berries

37. LEMON GELATIN DESSERT

INGREDIENTS:

- 3 1/3 cups = 800 ml filtered water
- 3 bags Lemon Zinger herbal tea
- 1/2 cup = 120 ml powdered erythritol
- 30 drops Lemon Twist stevia
- 3 tablespoons freshly squeezed juice from organic lemon
- 1 1/2 tablespoons unflavored grass-fed gelatin powder

METHOD:

1. Heat 3 cups (710 ml) of the water until boiling.
2. Add the teabags and the sweeteners. Let cool to room temperature and remove the tea bags, gently squeezing to save all the liquid.
3. Take the rest (1/3 cup ≈ 80 ml) of the water and pour it into a microwave safe cup.
4. Add the lemon juice. Sprinkle the gelatin powder on top.
5. Set for 10 minutes.
6. Heat the gelatin mixture in a microwave until steaming hot but not boiling. Mix to ensure that the entire gelatin is dissolved.
7. Pour the hot gelatin mixture into the tea mixture, constantly stirring.
8. Set aside.
9. Spray or brush gelatin molds with light olive oil. You can also use a silicone tube pan.
10. After the gelatin is dissolved in the tea mixture, pour the mixture into the gelatin molds or the silicone tube pan.
11. Refrigerate for 6 hours, or until set.
12. Before serving, rinse the bottom of the molds under hot, running water.
13. Notice that no dessert should get in touch with the hot water.

14. Carefully remove the gelatin from the molds: place a serving plate upside down on top of a mold.
15. Hold both the mold and the serving plate tightly together and quickly turn over the whole thing.
16. Remove extremely carefully the mold, ensuring that the gelatin comes out nicely and completely.
17. Repeat with the rest of the molds.
18. Decorate if you wish, and serve immediately.
19. Store the leftovers in the fridge.

38. STRAWBERRY COCONUT POPSICLES

INGREDIENTS:

- 1.25 cups Strawberries, fresh or frozen
- 1 tablespoon Liquid Stevia, or Local Honey
- 1 teaspoon Vanilla Extract
- ¾ cup Coconut Milk, from a can

METHOD:

1. Optional: Defrost frozen berries the night before.
2. Place the strawberries, vanilla extract, coconut milk and stevia or honey in a blender.
3. Blend ingredients until combined.
4. Pour into Popsicle molds (6X).
5. Freeze for at least 6 hours

39. CHOCOLATE BLACK FOREST TRIFLE

INGREDIENTS:

- 1 8 oz. package no-sugar-added low-fat chocolate cake mix
- 1 large sugar-free instant chocolate pudding mix
- 2 cups fat-free milk
- 1-pound fresh cherries (pitted), or frozen cherries, thaw and drain before preparing recipe.
- 2 cups thawed fat free dessert topping (cool Whip)
- Optional topping: unsweetened cocoa powder

METHOD:

1. Prepare cake mix according to directions on the package using the 8-inch square or round cake pan method.
2. Cool prepared cake for 10 minutes
3. Remove cake from pan and cut into ten 1-inch pieces.
4. Prepare the pudding while the cake bakes according to package directions but use 2 cups fat-free milk.
5. Cover prepared pudding and chill for 30 minutes.
6. A trifle is a layer, so you will need to layer the cake, cherries, and frozen topping into a 3-quart trifle bowl.
7. You can make less thick layers, or more thin layers.
8. Thin typically works best.
9. Continue to layer until you run out of cake and the final layer should be the frozen topping.
10. Sprinkle chocolate shavings or cocoa powder if desired.

40. LOW-SUGAR BROWNIES

INGREDIENTS:

- 3 tablespoon. Nutiva Organic Coconut Flour, sifted
- ¼ cup natural cocoa powder
- ¼ teaspoon sea salt 1 cup creamy almond butter, sunflower seed butter or macadamia nut butter
- 1 teaspoon organic vanilla extract
- 1 tsp. grass-fed gelatin
- 2 tablespoons Enjoy Life Dark Chocolate Morsels, melted
- 2 tablespoons Navitas Naturals Organic Palm Sugar (Coconut Sugar)
- 4 tablespoon Wholesome Sweeteners Organic Zero (Erythritol)
- ½ teaspoon baking soda
- 10 tablespoon filtered water
- 1 teaspoon liquid stevia (to taste)
- ½ teaspoon baking powder -

METHOD:

1. Preheat oven to 325 F.
2. Line the bottom of an 8-by-8 pan with unbleached parchment paper.
3. In a medium bowl, combine the coconut flour, coconut sugar, erythritol, cocoa powder, baking powder, baking soda and salt.
4. In a small bowl, add the water and sprinkle over the gelatin.
5. Let stand 5 minutes.
6. Add almond butter (or "nut" butter of choice), vanilla, stevia and melted chocolate.
7. Mix well using a hand-held mixer.
8. Pour in the dry ingredients and mix well to combine.

9. Spread brownie batter into prepared pan.
10. Transfer to oven and bake 30-35 minutes or until edges pull away and center is set.
11. If you like your brownies fudgy and moist inside, remove when center is still smoothly, at about 30 minutes.
12. Place on a wire rack to cool completely, then slice into squares.

CONCLUSION

I really hope you liked this book and all the recipes in it.

I would like to take this opportunity and thank you for purchasing my eBook.

It means a lot to me and I hope you'll find more books you like from my list above.

Please take a few minutes to leave a kind review on amazon, as it can help my brand grow and allow me to get more books out there each month.

Sincerely yours,

Katya.

Made in the USA
Monee, IL
02 January 2020